ABCs of
Classical Ballet

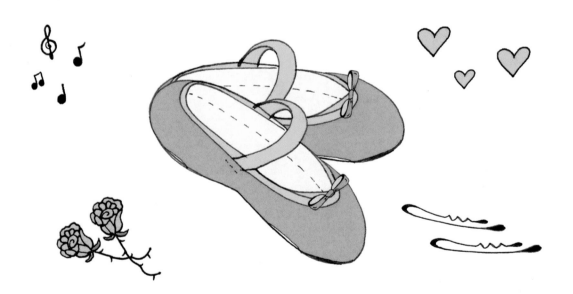

Written and Illustrated by Vanessa Salgado
with Donna Salgado

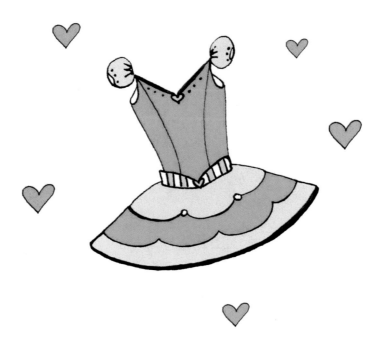

Published by Crafterina
ISBN 978-0-9886652-9-3
www.Crafterina.com

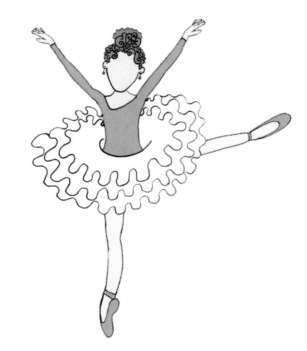

Arabesque

Bobby pin

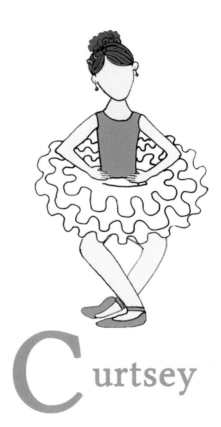

C urtsey

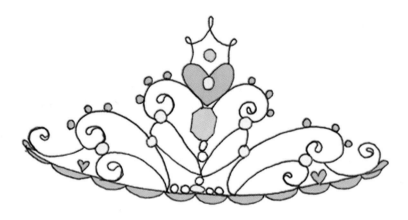

Diamond Tiara

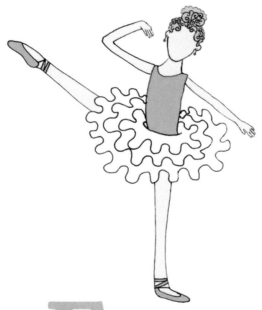

Extension

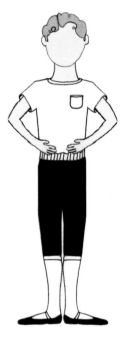

First Position

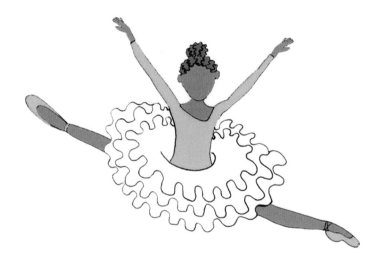

G rand Jeté

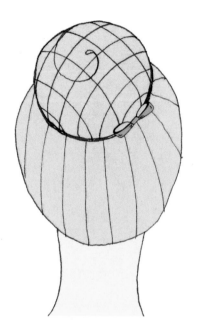

Hairnet

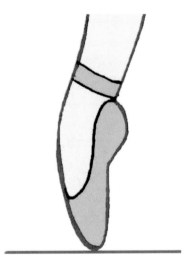

Instep

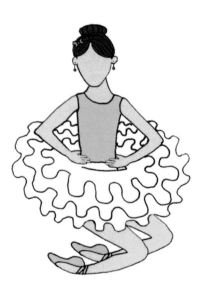

J ump

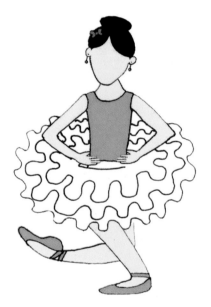

Kneel

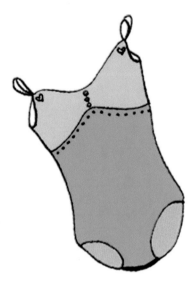

L eotard

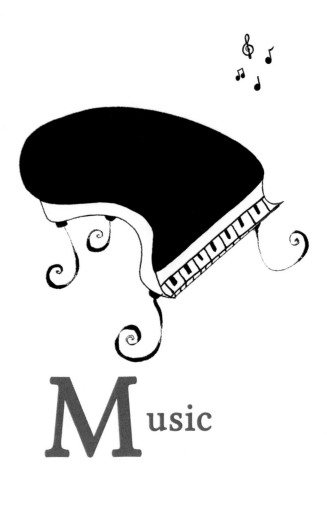

Music

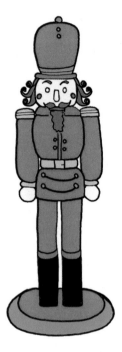

Nutcracker

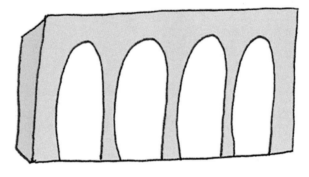

Opera House

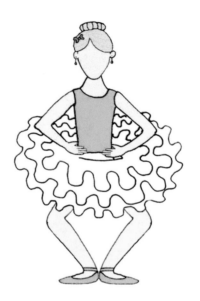

P lié

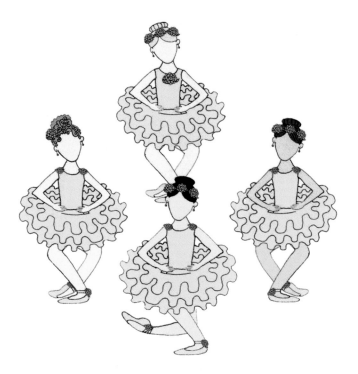

Pas de Quatre

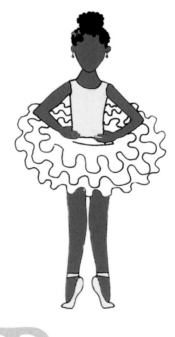

R elevé

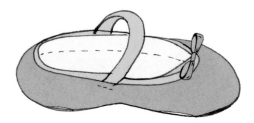

Ballet Slipper

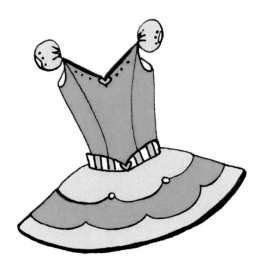

Tutu

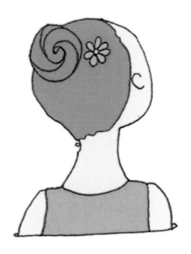

U pdo

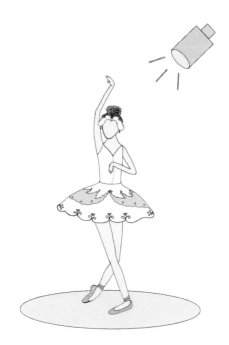

Variation

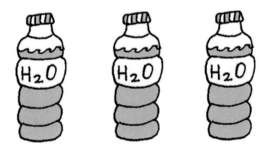

Water

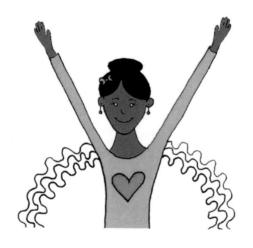

eXpression

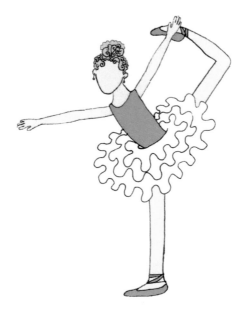

Yoga

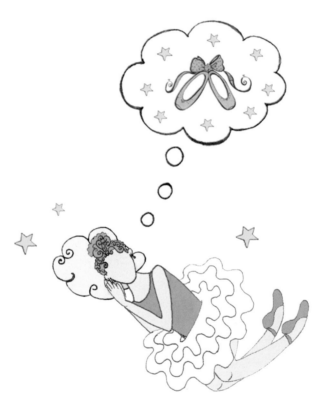

Z ZZZZZZ'S

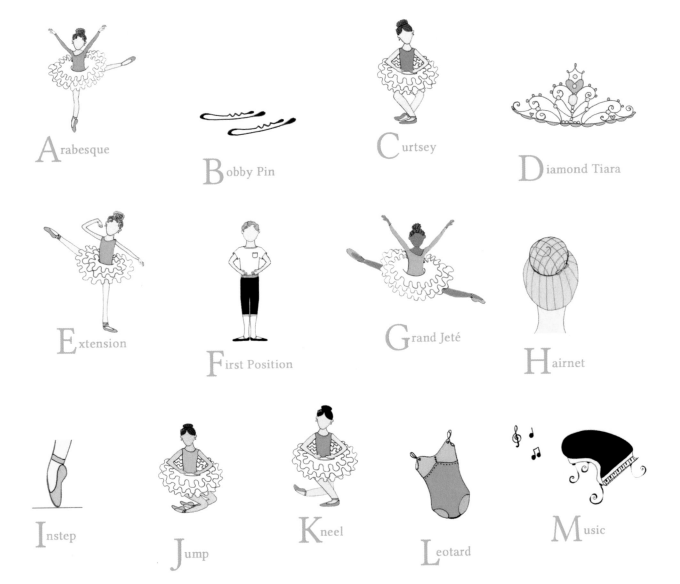

A rabesque

B obby Pin

C urtsey

D iamond Tiara

E xtension

F irst Position

G rand Jeté

H airnet

I nstep

J ump

K neel

L eotard

M usic

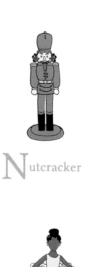

Nutcracker

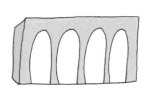

Opera House

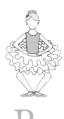

Plié

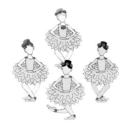

Pas de Quatre

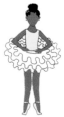

Relevé

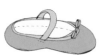

Ballet Slipper

Tutu

Updo

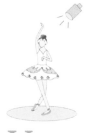

Variation

Water

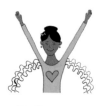

eXpression

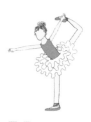

Yoga Stretch

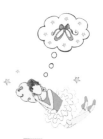

Zzzzzz's

Ballet Tips for Parents

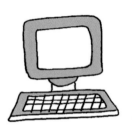

1. Research Teachers

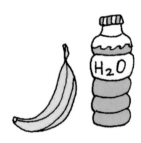

2. Pack Snacks

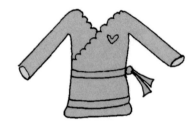

3. Bring a Sweater

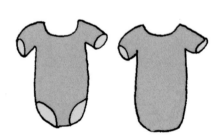

4. Front & Back of Leotard

5. Give Flowers at the Recital

How to Make a Ballet Bun

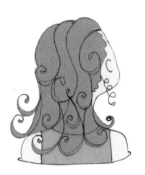

1. Brush Hair

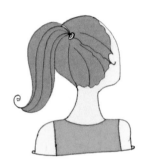

2. Pony Tail

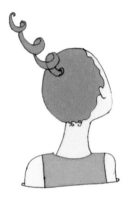

3. Twist

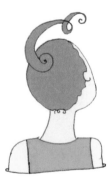

4. Pin as you Swirl

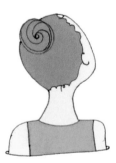

5. Add Bobby Pins

How to Prepare Ballet Slippers for Class

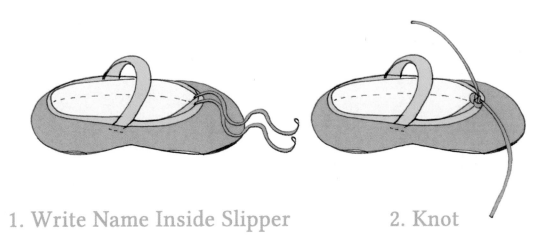

1. Write Name Inside Slipper

2. Knot

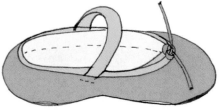

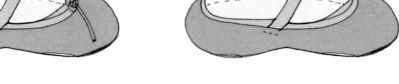

3. Trim

4. Tuck

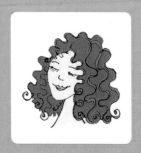

About the Author and Illustrator:
Vanessa Salgado is a Professional Dancer and Visual Artist based out of New York City.
She has taught creative movement and foundational ballet classes to many little dancers
throughout Manhattan.

Vanessa is a graduate of the world famous Alvin Ailey/Fordham University BFA Program at Lincoln Center.
She also holds a Certification in Dance Education from the Dance Education Laboratory
at the NY 92nd St. Y Harkness Dance Center.

Her earliest memories involve story time with her dad, creating with her mom after school,
and attending weekend ballet class alongside her sister, Donna.

Her interests in visual art revealed themselves wholeheartedly in high school
as she simultaneously trained vigorously for the professional dance world.
As she transitioned into her college days and now into her professional life,
her incessant doodles and crafting have remained a source of wonder for all those around her.

For more information about Vanessa, please visit www.VanessaSalgado.com.
Please visit www.Crafterina.com for children's crafts and dance resources.

www.Crafterina.com

Made in the USA
Coppell, TX
13 July 2023

19088521R00021